@ Safe Haven Sobriety

This Planner Belongs To

Name:	
Phone:	
E-Mail:	
Address:	

Sponsor

Name:	
Phone:	

Emergency Contact Information

Name:	
Phone:	
E-Mail:	

2020   One Day at a Time

@ SAFE HAVEN SOBRIETY

DAILY INVENTORY

Did I pray to know and follow God's will today?

What progress did I make?

What weaknesses do I need to surrender to God?

In what ways was I kind and loving?

Was I able to "let go and let God?"

Do I need to make amends to anyone?

Did faith or fear control my thoughts?

Am I taking care of myself physically, emotionally, and spiritually?

What am I grateful for today?

COMMENTS

@ Safe Haven Sobriety

PERSONAL NOTES

PERSONAL

RELATIONS

SPIRITUAL

@ SAFE HAVEN SOBRIETY

DAILY INVENTORY

| Did I pray to know and follow God's will today? |

| What progress did I make? |

| What weaknesses do I need to surrender to God? |

| In what ways was I kind and loving? |

| Was I able to "let go and let God?" |

| Do I need to make amends to anyone? |

| Did faith or fear control my thoughts? |

| Am I taking care of myself physically, emotionally, and spiritually? |

| What am I grateful for today? |

COMMENTS

_____

_____

@ Safe Haven Sobriety

PERSONAL NOTES

PERSONAL

RELATIONS

SPIRITUAL

@ SAFE HAVEN SOBRIETY

DAILY INVENTORY

Did I pray to know and follow God's will today?

What progress did I make?

What weaknesses do I need to surrender to God?

In what ways was I kind and loving?

Was I able to "let go and let God?"

Do I need to make amends to anyone?

Did faith or fear control my thoughts?

Am I taking care of myself physically, emotionally, and spiritually?

What am I grateful for today?

COMMENTS

@ Safe Haven Sobriety

PERSONAL NOTES

PERSONAL

RELATIONS

SPIRITUAL

@ SAFE HAVEN SOBRIETY

DAILY INVENTORY

Did I pray to know and follow God's will today?	

What progress did I make?	

What weaknesses do I need to surrender to God?	

In what ways was I kind and loving?	

Was I able to "let go and let God?"	

Do I need to make amends to anyone?	

Did faith or fear control my thoughts?	

Am I taking care of myself physically, emotionally, and spiritually?	

What am I grateful for today?	

COMMENTS

_____

_____

@ Safe Haven Sobriety

PERSONAL NOTES

PERSONAL

RELATIONS

SPIRITUAL

@ SAFE HAVEN SOBRIETY

DAILY INVENTORY

Did I pray to know and follow God's will today?

What progress did I make?

What weaknesses do I need to surrender to God?

In what ways was I kind and loving?

Was I able to "let go and let God?"

Do I need to make amends to anyone?

Did faith or fear control my thoughts?

Am I taking care of myself physically, emotionally, and spiritually?

What am I grateful for today?

COMMENTS

@ SAFE HAVEN SOBRIETY

PERSONAL NOTES

PERSONAL

RELATIONS

SPIRITUAL

@ S̲AFE H̲AVEN S̲OBRIETY

DAILY INVENTORY

Did I pray to know and follow God's will today?

What progress did I make?

What weaknesses do I need to surrender to God?

In what ways was I kind and loving?

Was I able to "let go and let God?"

Do I need to make amends to anyone?

Did faith or fear control my thoughts?

Am I taking care of myself physically, emotionally, and spiritually?

What am I grateful for today?

COMMENTS

@ SAFE HAVEN SOBRIETY

PERSONAL NOTES

PERSONAL

RELATIONS

SPIRITUAL

@ SAFE HAVEN SOBRIETY

DAILY INVENTORY

Did I pray to know and follow God's will today?	

What progress did I make?	

What weaknesses do I need to surrender to God?	

In what ways was I kind and loving?	

Was I able to "let go and let God?"	

Do I need to make amends to anyone?	

Did faith or fear control my thoughts?	

Am I taking care of myself physically, emotionally, and spiritually?	

What am I grateful for today?	

COMMENTS

_____

_____

@ Safe Haven Sobriety

PERSONAL NOTES

PERSONAL

RELATIONS

SPIRITUAL

@ SAFE HAVEN SOBRIETY

DAILY INVENTORY

Did I pray to know and follow God's will today?

What progress did I make?

What weaknesses do I need to surrender to God?

In what ways was I kind and loving?

Was I able to "let go and let God?"

Do I need to make amends to anyone?

Did faith or fear control my thoughts?

Am I taking care of myself physically, emotionally, and spiritually?

What am I grateful for today?

COMMENTS

@ Safe Haven Sobriety

PERSONAL NOTES

PERSONAL

RELATIONS

SPIRITUAL

@ SAFE HAVEN SOBRIETY

DAILY INVENTORY

Did I pray to know and follow God's will today?

What progress did I make?

What weaknesses do I need to surrender to God?

In what ways was I kind and loving?

Was I able to "let go and let God?"

Do I need to make amends to anyone?

Did faith or fear control my thoughts?

Am I taking care of myself physically, emotionally, and spiritually?

What am I grateful for today?

COMMENTS

@ Safe Haven Sobriety

PERSONAL NOTES

PERSONAL

RELATIONS

SPIRITUAL

@ SAFE HAVEN SOBRIETY

DAILY INVENTORY

| Did I pray to know and follow God's will today? | |

| What progress did I make? | |

| What weaknesses do I need to surrender to God? | |

| In what ways was I kind and loving? | |

| Was I able to "let go and let God?" | |

| Do I need to make amends to anyone? | |

| Did faith or fear control my thoughts? | |

| Am I taking care of myself physically, emotionally, and spiritually? | |

| What am I grateful for today? | |

COMMENTS

_____

_____

_____

@ Safe Haven Sobriety

PERSONAL NOTES

PERSONAL

RELATIONS

SPIRITUAL

@ SAFE HAVEN SOBRIETY

DAILY INVENTORY

Did I pray to know and follow God's will today?	

What progress did I make?	

What weaknesses do I need to surrender to God?	

In what ways was I kind and loving?	

Was I able to "let go and let God?"	

Do I need to make amends to anyone?	

Did faith or fear control my thoughts?	

Am I taking care of myself physically, emotionally, and spiritually?	

What am I grateful for today?	

COMMENTS

_____

_____

@ Safe Haven Sobriety

PERSONAL NOTES

PERSONAL

RELATIONS

SPIRITUAL

@ SAFE HAVEN SOBRIETY

DAILY INVENTORY

Did I pray to know and follow God's will today?

What progress did I make?

What weaknesses do I need to surrender to God?

In what ways was I kind and loving?

Was I able to "let go and let God?"

Do I need to make amends to anyone?

Did faith or fear control my thoughts?

Am I taking care of myself physically, emotionally, and spiritually?

What am I grateful for today?

COMMENTS

@ Safe Haven Sobriety

PERSONAL NOTES

PERSONAL

RELATIONS

SPIRITUAL

@ SAFE HAVEN SOBRIETY

DAILY INVENTORY

Did I pray to know and follow God's will today?	

What progress did I make?	

What weaknesses do I need to surrender to God?	

In what ways was I kind and loving?	

Was I able to "let go and let God?"	

Do I need to make amends to anyone?	

Did faith or fear control my thoughts?	

Am I taking care of myself physically, emotionally, and spiritually?	

What am I grateful for today?	

COMMENTS

_____

_____

@ Safe Haven Sobriety

PERSONAL NOTES

PERSONAL

RELATIONS

SPIRITUAL

@ SAFE HAVEN SOBRIETY

DAILY INVENTORY

Did I pray to know and follow God's will today?

What progress did I make?

What weaknesses do I need to surrender to God?

In what ways was I kind and loving?

Was I able to "let go and let God?"

Do I need to make amends to anyone?

Did faith or fear control my thoughts?

Am I taking care of myself physically, emotionally, and spiritually?

What am I grateful for today?

COMMENTS

@ Safe Haven Sobriety

PERSONAL NOTES

PERSONAL

RELATIONS

SPIRITUAL

@ SAFE HAVEN SOBRIETY

DAILY INVENTORY

| Did I pray to know and follow God's will today? | |

| What progress did I make? | |

| What weaknesses do I need to surrender to God? | |

| In what ways was I kind and loving? | |

| Was I able to "let go and let God?" | |

| Do I need to make amends to anyone? | |

| Did faith or fear control my thoughts? | |

| Am I taking care of myself physically, emotionally, and spiritually? | |

| What am I grateful for today? | |

COMMENTS

@ Safe Haven Sobriety

PERSONAL NOTES

PERSONAL

RELATIONS

SPIRITUAL

@ SAFE HAVEN SOBRIETY

DAILY INVENTORY

Did I pray to know and follow God's will today?

What progress did I make?

What weaknesses do I need to surrender to God?

In what ways was I kind and loving?

Was I able to "let go and let God?"

Do I need to make amends to anyone?

Did faith or fear control my thoughts?

Am I taking care of myself physically, emotionally, and spiritually?

What am I grateful for today?

COMMENTS

@ SAFE HAVEN SOBRIETY

PERSONAL NOTES

PERSONAL

RELATIONS

SPIRITUAL

@ SAFE HAVEN SOBRIETY

DAILY INVENTORY

Did I pray to know and follow God's will today?

What progress did I make?

What weaknesses do I need to surrender to God?

In what ways was I kind and loving?

Was I able to "let go and let God?"

Do I need to make amends to anyone?

Did faith or fear control my thoughts?

Am I taking care of myself physically, emotionally, and spiritually?

What am I grateful for today?

COMMENTS

@ Safe Haven Sobriety

PERSONAL NOTES

PERSONAL

RELATIONS

SPIRITUAL

@ SAFE HAVEN SOBRIETY

DAILY INVENTORY

| Did I pray to know and follow God's will today? | |

| What progress did I make? | |

| What weaknesses do I need to surrender to God? | |

| In what ways was I kind and loving? | |

| Was I able to "let go and let God?" | |

| Do I need to make amends to anyone? | |

| Did faith or fear control my thoughts? | |

| Am I taking care of myself physically, emotionally, and spiritually? | |

| What am I grateful for today? | |

COMMENTS

@ Safe Haven Sobriety

PERSONAL NOTES

PERSONAL

RELATIONS

SPIRITUAL

@ SAFE HAVEN SOBRIETY

DAILY INVENTORY

Did I pray to know and follow God's will today?	

What progress did I make?	

What weaknesses do I need to surrender to God?	

In what ways was I kind and loving?	

Was I able to "let go and let God?"	

Do I need to make amends to anyone?	

Did faith or fear control my thoughts?	

Am I taking care of myself physically, emotionally, and spiritually?	

What am I grateful for today?	

COMMENTS

_____

_____

@ Safe Haven Sobriety

PERSONAL NOTES

PERSONAL

RELATIONS

SPIRITUAL

@ SAFE HAVEN SOBRIETY

DAILY INVENTORY

Did I pray to know and follow God's will today?	

What progress did I make?	

What weaknesses do I need to surrender to God?	

In what ways was I kind and loving?	

Was I able to "let go and let God?"	

Do I need to make amends to anyone?	

Did faith or fear control my thoughts?	

Am I taking care of myself physically, emotionally, and spiritually?	

What am I grateful for today?	

COMMENTS

_____

_____

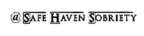

PERSONAL NOTES

PERSONAL

RELATIONS

SPIRITUAL

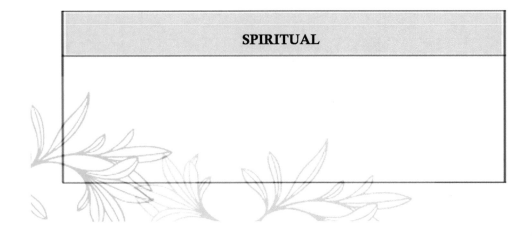

@ SAFE HAVEN SOBRIETY

DAILY INVENTORY

Did I pray to know and follow God's will today?

What progress did I make?

What weaknesses do I need to surrender to God?

In what ways was I kind and loving?

Was I able to "let go and let God?"

Do I need to make amends to anyone?

Did faith or fear control my thoughts?

Am I taking care of myself physically, emotionally, and spiritually?

What am I grateful for today?

COMMENTS

_____

_____

_____

@ Safe Haven Sobriety

PERSONAL NOTES

PERSONAL

RELATIONS

SPIRITUAL

@ SAFE HAVEN SOBRIETY

DAILY INVENTORY

Did I pray to know and follow God's will today?

What progress did I make?

What weaknesses do I need to surrender to God?

In what ways was I kind and loving?

Was I able to "let go and let God?"

Do I need to make amends to anyone?

Did faith or fear control my thoughts?

Am I taking care of myself physically, emotionally, and spiritually?

What am I grateful for today?

COMMENTS

@ SAFE HAVEN SOBRIETY

PERSONAL NOTES

PERSONAL

RELATIONS

SPIRITUAL

@ SAFE HAVEN SOBRIETY

DAILY INVENTORY

| Did I pray to know and follow God's will today? | |

| What progress did I make? | |

| What weaknesses do I need to surrender to God? | |

| In what ways was I kind and loving? | |

| Was I able to "let go and let God?" | |

| Do I need to make amends to anyone? | |

| Did faith or fear control my thoughts? | |

| Am I taking care of myself physically, emotionally, and spiritually? | |

| What am I grateful for today? | |

COMMENTS

_____

_____

@ SAFE HAVEN SOBRIETY

PERSONAL NOTES

PERSONAL

RELATIONS

SPIRITUAL

@ S̲AFE H̲AVEN S̲OBRIETY

DAILY INVENTORY

| Did I pray to know and follow God's will today? | |

| What progress did I make? | |

| What weaknesses do I need to surrender to God? | |

| In what ways was I kind and loving? | |

| Was I able to "let go and let God?" | |

| Do I need to make amends to anyone? | |

| Did faith or fear control my thoughts? | |

| Am I taking care of myself physically, emotionally, and spiritually? | |

| What am I grateful for today? | |

COMMENTS

@ SAFE HAVEN SOBRIETY

PERSONAL NOTES

PERSONAL

RELATIONS

SPIRITUAL

@ SAFE HAVEN SOBRIETY

DAILY INVENTORY

| Did I pray to know and follow God's will today? | |

| What progress did I make? | |

| What weaknesses do I need to surrender to God? | |

| In what ways was I kind and loving? | |

| Was I able to "let go and let God?" | |

| Do I need to make amends to anyone? | |

| Did faith or fear control my thoughts? | |

| Am I taking care of myself physically, emotionally, and spiritually? | |

| What am I grateful for today? | |

COMMENTS

@ Safe Haven Sobriety

PERSONAL NOTES

PERSONAL

RELATIONS

SPIRITUAL

@ SAFE HAVEN SOBRIETY

DAILY INVENTORY

Did I pray to know and follow God's will today?	

What progress did I make?	

What weaknesses do I need to surrender to God?	

In what ways was I kind and loving?	

Was I able to "let go and let God?"	

Do I need to make amends to anyone?	

Did faith or fear control my thoughts?	

Am I taking care of myself physically, emotionally, and spiritually?	

What am I grateful for today?	

COMMENTS

_____

_____

@ Safe Haven Sobriety

PERSONAL NOTES

PERSONAL

RELATIONS

SPIRITUAL

@ SAFE HAVEN SOBRIETY

DAILY INVENTORY

Did I pray to know and follow God's will today?	

What progress did I make?	

What weaknesses do I need to surrender to God?	

In what ways was I kind and loving?	

Was I able to "let go and let God?"	

Do I need to make amends to anyone?	

Did faith or fear control my thoughts?	

Am I taking care of myself physically, emotionally, and spiritually?	

What am I grateful for today?	

COMMENTS

_____

_____

@ Safe Haven Sobriety

PERSONAL NOTES

PERSONAL

RELATIONS

SPIRITUAL

@ SAFE HAVEN SOBRIETY

DAILY INVENTORY

Did I pray to know and follow God's will today?

What progress did I make?

What weaknesses do I need to surrender to God?

In what ways was I kind and loving?

Was I able to "let go and let God?"

Do I need to make amends to anyone?

Did faith or fear control my thoughts?

Am I taking care of myself physically, emotionally, and spiritually?

What am I grateful for today?

COMMENTS

@ Safe Haven Sobriety

PERSONAL NOTES

PERSONAL

RELATIONS

SPIRITUAL

@ SAFE HAVEN SOBRIETY

DAILY INVENTORY

Did I pray to know and follow God's will today?

What progress did I make?

What weaknesses do I need to surrender to God?

In what ways was I kind and loving?

Was I able to "let go and let God?"

Do I need to make amends to anyone?

Did faith or fear control my thoughts?

Am I taking care of myself physically, emotionally, and spiritually?

What am I grateful for today?

COMMENTS

@ Safe Haven Sobriety

PERSONAL NOTES

PERSONAL

RELATIONS

SPIRITUAL

@ S̲AFE H̲AVEN S̲OBRIETY

DAILY INVENTORY

Did I pray to know and follow God's will today?

What progress did I make?

What weaknesses do I need to surrender to God?

In what ways was I kind and loving?

Was I able to "let go and let God?"

Do I need to make amends to anyone?

Did faith or fear control my thoughts?

Am I taking care of myself physically, emotionally, and spiritually?

What am I grateful for today?

COMMENTS

@ SAFE HAVEN SOBRIETY

PERSONAL NOTES

PERSONAL

RELATIONS

SPIRITUAL

@ SAFE HAVEN SOBRIETY

DAILY INVENTORY

Did I pray to know and follow God's will today?	

What progress did I make?	

What weaknesses do I need to surrender to God?	

In what ways was I kind and loving?	

Was I able to "let go and let God?"	

Do I need to make amends to anyone?	

Did faith or fear control my thoughts?	

Am I taking care of myself physically, emotionally, and spiritually?	

What am I grateful for today?	

COMMENTS

_____

_____

@ Safe Haven Sobriety

PERSONAL NOTES

PERSONAL

RELATIONS

SPIRITUAL

@ SAFE HAVEN SOBRIETY

DAILY INVENTORY

| Did I pray to know and follow God's will today? | |

| What progress did I make? | |

| What weaknesses do I need to surrender to God? | |

| In what ways was I kind and loving? | |

| Was I able to "let go and let God?" | |

| Do I need to make amends to anyone? | |

| Did faith or fear control my thoughts? | |

| Am I taking care of myself physically, emotionally, and spiritually? | |

| What am I grateful for today? | |

COMMENTS

@ Safe Haven Sobriety

PERSONAL NOTES

PERSONAL

RELATIONS

SPIRITUAL

@ SAFE HAVEN SOBRIETY

DAILY INVENTORY

| Did I pray to know and follow God's will today? | |

| What progress did I make? | |

| What weaknesses do I need to surrender to God? | |

| In what ways was I kind and loving? | |

| Was I able to "let go and let God?" | |

| Do I need to make amends to anyone? | |

| Did faith or fear control my thoughts? | |

| Am I taking care of myself physically, emotionally, and spiritually? | |

| What am I grateful for today? | |

COMMENTS

_____

_____

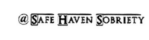

PERSONAL NOTES

PERSONAL

RELATIONS

SPIRITUAL

@ **S**AFE **H**AVEN **S**OBRIETY

DAILY INVENTORY

Did I pray to know and follow God's will today?	

What progress did I make?	

What weaknesses do I need to surrender to God?	

In what ways was I kind and loving?	

Was I able to "let go and let God?"	

Do I need to make amends to anyone?	

Did faith or fear control my thoughts?	

Am I taking care of myself physically, emotionally, and spiritually?	

What am I grateful for today?	

COMMENTS

_____

_____

@ Safe Haven Sobriety

PERSONAL NOTES

PERSONAL

RELATIONS

SPIRITUAL

@ **S**AFE **H**AVEN **S**OBRIETY

DAILY INVENTORY

Did I pray to know and follow God's will today?	

What progress did I make?	

What weaknesses do I need to surrender to God?	

In what ways was I kind and loving?	

Was I able to "let go and let God?"	

Do I need to make amends to anyone?	

Did faith or fear control my thoughts?	

Am I taking care of myself physically, emotionally, and spiritually?	

What am I grateful for today?	

COMMENTS

_____

_____

@ Safe Haven Sobriety

PERSONAL NOTES

PERSONAL

RELATIONS

SPIRITUAL

@ SAFE HAVEN SOBRIETY

DAILY INVENTORY

| Did I pray to know and follow God's will today? | |

| What progress did I make? | |

| What weaknesses do I need to surrender to God? | |

| In what ways was I kind and loving? | |

| Was I able to "let go and let God?" | |

| Do I need to make amends to anyone? | |

| Did faith or fear control my thoughts? | |

| Am I taking care of myself physically, emotionally, and spiritually? | |

| What am I grateful for today? | |

COMMENTS

_____

_____

@ Safe Haven Sobriety

PERSONAL NOTES

PERSONAL

RELATIONS

SPIRITUAL

@ SAFE HAVEN SOBRIETY

DAILY INVENTORY

Did I pray to know and follow God's will today?

What progress did I make?

What weaknesses do I need to surrender to God?

In what ways was I kind and loving?

Was I able to "let go and let God?"

Do I need to make amends to anyone?

Did faith or fear control my thoughts?

Am I taking care of myself physically, emotionally, and spiritually?

What am I grateful for today?

COMMENTS

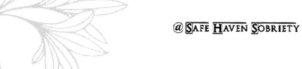

PERSONAL NOTES

PERSONAL

RELATIONS

SPIRITUAL

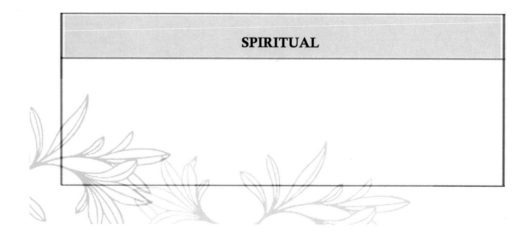

@ SAFE HAVEN SOBRIETY

DAILY INVENTORY

| Did I pray to know and follow God's will today? | |

| What progress did I make? | |

| What weaknesses do I need to surrender to God? | |

| In what ways was I kind and loving? | |

| Was I able to "let go and let God?" | |

| Do I need to make amends to anyone? | |

| Did faith or fear control my thoughts? | |

| Am I taking care of myself physically, emotionally, and spiritually? | |

| What am I grateful for today? | |

COMMENTS

@ Safe Haven Sobriety

PERSONAL NOTES

PERSONAL

RELATIONS

SPIRITUAL

@ SAFE HAVEN SOBRIETY

DAILY INVENTORY

| Did I pray to know and follow God's will today? | |

| What progress did I make? | |

| What weaknesses do I need to surrender to God? | |

| In what ways was I kind and loving? | |

| Was I able to "let go and let God?" | |

| Do I need to make amends to anyone? | |

| Did faith or fear control my thoughts? | |

| Am I taking care of myself physically, emotionally, and spiritually? | |

| What am I grateful for today? | |

COMMENTS

PERSONAL NOTES

PERSONAL

RELATIONS

SPIRITUAL

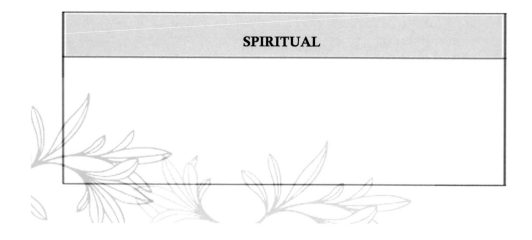

@ SAFE HAVEN SOBRIETY

DAILY INVENTORY

Did I pray to know and follow God's will today?

What progress did I make?

What weaknesses do I need to surrender to God?

In what ways was I kind and loving?

Was I able to "let go and let God?"

Do I need to make amends to anyone?

Did faith or fear control my thoughts?

Am I taking care of myself physically, emotionally, and spiritually?

What am I grateful for today?

COMMENTS

@ Safe Haven Sobriety

PERSONAL NOTES

PERSONAL

RELATIONS

SPIRITUAL

@ SAFE HAVEN SOBRIETY

DAILY INVENTORY

Did I pray to know and follow God's will today?

What progress did I make?

What weaknesses do I need to surrender to God?

In what ways was I kind and loving?

Was I able to "let go and let God?"

Do I need to make amends to anyone?

Did faith or fear control my thoughts?

Am I taking care of myself physically, emotionally, and spiritually?

What am I grateful for today?

COMMENTS

@ SAFE HAVEN SOBRIETY

PERSONAL NOTES

PERSONAL

RELATIONS

SPIRITUAL

@ S̲AFE H̲AVEN S̲OBRIETY

DAILY INVENTORY

Did I pray to know and follow God's will today?

What progress did I make?

What weaknesses do I need to surrender to God?

In what ways was I kind and loving?

Was I able to "let go and let God?"

Do I need to make amends to anyone?

Did faith or fear control my thoughts?

Am I taking care of myself physically, emotionally, and spiritually?

What am I grateful for today?

COMMENTS

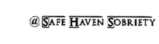

PERSONAL NOTES

PERSONAL

RELATIONS

SPIRITUAL

@ SAFE HAVEN SOBRIETY

DAILY INVENTORY

| Did I pray to know and follow God's will today? | |

| What progress did I make? | |

| What weaknesses do I need to surrender to God? | |

| In what ways was I kind and loving? | |

| Was I able to "let go and let God?" | |

| Do I need to make amends to anyone? | |

| Did faith or fear control my thoughts? | |

| Am I taking care of myself physically, emotionally, and spiritually? | |

| What am I grateful for today? | |

COMMENTS

_____

_____

@ Safe Haven Sobriety

PERSONAL NOTES

PERSONAL

RELATIONS

SPIRITUAL

@ SAFE HAVEN SOBRIETY

DAILY INVENTORY

Did I pray to know and follow God's will today?	

What progress did I make?	

What weaknesses do I need to surrender to God?	

In what ways was I kind and loving?	

Was I able to "let go and let God?"	

Do I need to make amends to anyone?	

Did faith or fear control my thoughts?	

Am I taking care of myself physically, emotionally, and spiritually?	

What am I grateful for today?	

COMMENTS

_____

_____

@ Safe Haven Sobriety

PERSONAL NOTES

PERSONAL

RELATIONS

SPIRITUAL

@ SAFE HAVEN SOBRIETY

DAILY INVENTORY

Did I pray to know and follow God's will today?

What progress did I make?

What weaknesses do I need to surrender to God?

In what ways was I kind and loving?

Was I able to "let go and let God?"

Do I need to make amends to anyone?

Did faith or fear control my thoughts?

Am I taking care of myself physically, emotionally, and spiritually?

What am I grateful for today?

COMMENTS

@ SAFE HAVEN SOBRIETY

PERSONAL NOTES

PERSONAL

RELATIONS

SPIRITUAL

@ SAFE HAVEN SOBRIETY

DAILY INVENTORY

| Did I pray to know and follow God's will today? | |

| What progress did I make? | |

| What weaknesses do I need to surrender to God? | |

| In what ways was I kind and loving? | |

| Was I able to "let go and let God?" | |

| Do I need to make amends to anyone? | |

| Did faith or fear control my thoughts? | |

| Am I taking care of myself physically, emotionally, and spiritually? | |

| What am I grateful for today? | |

COMMENTS

_____

_____

@ Safe Haven Sobriety

PERSONAL NOTES

PERSONAL

RELATIONS

SPIRITUAL

@ SAFE HAVEN SOBRIETY

DAILY INVENTORY

Did I pray to know and follow God's will today?	

What progress did I make?	

What weaknesses do I need to surrender to God?	

In what ways was I kind and loving?	

Was I able to "let go and let God?"	

Do I need to make amends to anyone?	

Did faith or fear control my thoughts?	

Am I taking care of myself physically, emotionally, and spiritually?	

What am I grateful for today?	

COMMENTS

_____

_____

@ SAFE HAVEN SOBRIETY

PERSONAL NOTES

PERSONAL

RELATIONS

SPIRITUAL

@ SAFE HAVEN SOBRIETY

DAILY INVENTORY

| Did I pray to know and follow God's will today? | |

| What progress did I make? | |

| What weaknesses do I need to surrender to God? | |

| In what ways was I kind and loving? | |

| Was I able to "let go and let God?" | |

| Do I need to make amends to anyone? | |

| Did faith or fear control my thoughts? | |

| Am I taking care of myself physically, emotionally, and spiritually? | |

| What am I grateful for today? | |

COMMENTS

@ Safe Haven Sobriety

PERSONAL NOTES

PERSONAL

RELATIONS

SPIRITUAL

@ SAFE HAVEN SOBRIETY

DAILY INVENTORY

Did I pray to know and follow God's will today?

What progress did I make?

What weaknesses do I need to surrender to God?

In what ways was I kind and loving?

Was I able to "let go and let God?"

Do I need to make amends to anyone?

Did faith or fear control my thoughts?

Am I taking care of myself physically, emotionally, and spiritually?

What am I grateful for today?

COMMENTS
_____
_____

@ Safe Haven Sobriety

PERSONAL NOTES

PERSONAL

RELATIONS

SPIRITUAL

@ SAFE HAVEN SOBRIETY

DAILY INVENTORY

Did I pray to know and follow God's will today?

What progress did I make?

What weaknesses do I need to surrender to God?

In what ways was I kind and loving?

Was I able to "let go and let God?"

Do I need to make amends to anyone?

Did faith or fear control my thoughts?

Am I taking care of myself physically, emotionally, and spiritually?

What am I grateful for today?

COMMENTS

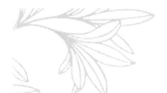

PERSONAL NOTES

PERSONAL

RELATIONS

SPIRITUAL

@ SAFE HAVEN SOBRIETY

DAILY INVENTORY

| Did I pray to know and follow God's will today? | |

| What progress did I make? | |

| What weaknesses do I need to surrender to God? | |

| In what ways was I kind and loving? | |

| Was I able to "let go and let God?" | |

| Do I need to make amends to anyone? | |

| Did faith or fear control my thoughts? | |

| Am I taking care of myself physically, emotionally, and spiritually? | |

| What am I grateful for today? | |

COMMENTS

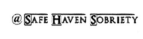

PERSONAL NOTES

PERSONAL

RELATIONS

SPIRITUAL

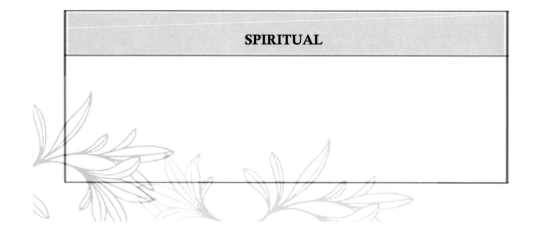

@ SAFE HAVEN SOBRIETY

DAILY INVENTORY

Did I pray to know and follow God's will today?

What progress did I make?

What weaknesses do I need to surrender to God?

In what ways was I kind and loving?

Was I able to "let go and let God?"

Do I need to make amends to anyone?

Did faith or fear control my thoughts?

Am I taking care of myself physically, emotionally, and spiritually?

What am I grateful for today?

COMMENTS

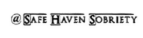

PERSONAL NOTES

PERSONAL

RELATIONS

SPIRITUAL

@ SAFE HAVEN SOBRIETY

DAILY INVENTORY

Did I pray to know and follow God's will today?	

What progress did I make?	

What weaknesses do I need to surrender to God?	

In what ways was I kind and loving?	

Was I able to "let go and let God?"	

Do I need to make amends to anyone?	

Did faith or fear control my thoughts?	

Am I taking care of myself physically, emotionally, and spiritually?	

What am I grateful for today?	

COMMENTS

_____

_____

@ Safe Haven Sobriety

PERSONAL NOTES

PERSONAL

RELATIONS

SPIRITUAL

@ SAFE HAVEN SOBRIETY

DAILY INVENTORY

Did I pray to know and follow God's will today?

What progress did I make?

What weaknesses do I need to surrender to God?

In what ways was I kind and loving?

Was I able to "let go and let God?"

Do I need to make amends to anyone?

Did faith or fear control my thoughts?

Am I taking care of myself physically, emotionally, and spiritually?

What am I grateful for today?

COMMENTS

@ SAFE HAVEN SOBRIETY

PERSONAL NOTES

PERSONAL

RELATIONS

SPIRITUAL

@ SAFE HAVEN SOBRIETY

DAILY INVENTORY

| Did I pray to know and follow God's will today? | |

| What progress did I make? | |

| What weaknesses do I need to surrender to God? | |

| In what ways was I kind and loving? | |

| Was I able to "let go and let God?" | |

| Do I need to make amends to anyone? | |

| Did faith or fear control my thoughts? | |

| Am I taking care of myself physically, emotionally, and spiritually? | |

| What am I grateful for today? | |

COMMENTS

_____

_____

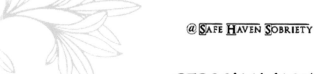

PERSONAL NOTES

PERSONAL

RELATIONS

SPIRITUAL

@ SAFE HAVEN SOBRIETY

DAILY INVENTORY

| Did I pray to know and follow God's will today? | |

| What progress did I make? | |

| What weaknesses do I need to surrender to God? | |

| In what ways was I kind and loving? | |

| Was I able to "let go and let God?" | |

| Do I need to make amends to anyone? | |

| Did faith or fear control my thoughts? | |

| Am I taking care of myself physically, emotionally, and spiritually? | |

| What am I grateful for today? | |

COMMENTS

_____

_____

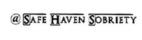

PERSONAL NOTES

PERSONAL

RELATIONS

SPIRITUAL

@ SAFE HAVEN SOBRIETY

DAILY INVENTORY

Did I pray to know and follow God's will today?	
What progress did I make?	
What weaknesses do I need to surrender to God?	
In what ways was I kind and loving?	
Was I able to "let go and let God?"	
Do I need to make amends to anyone?	
Did faith or fear control my thoughts?	
Am I taking care of myself physically, emotionally, and spiritually?	
What am I grateful for today?	

COMMENTS

_____

_____

@ Safe Haven Sobriety

PERSONAL NOTES

PERSONAL

RELATIONS

SPIRITUAL

@ SAFE HAVEN SOBRIETY

DAILY INVENTORY

| Did I pray to know and follow God's will today? | |

| What progress did I make? | |

| What weaknesses do I need to surrender to God? | |

| In what ways was I kind and loving? | |

| Was I able to "let go and let God?" | |

| Do I need to make amends to anyone? | |

| Did faith or fear control my thoughts? | |

| Am I taking care of myself physically, emotionally, and spiritually? | |

| What am I grateful for today? | |

COMMENTS

_____

_____

@ Safe Haven Sobriety

PERSONAL NOTES

PERSONAL

RELATIONS

SPIRITUAL

@ S̲afe H̲aven S̲obriety

DAILY INVENTORY

Did I pray to know and follow God's will today?	

What progress did I make?	

What weaknesses do I need to surrender to God?	

In what ways was I kind and loving?	

Was I able to "let go and let God?"	

Do I need to make amends to anyone?	

Did faith or fear control my thoughts?	

Am I taking care of myself physically, emotionally, and spiritually?	

What am I grateful for today?	

COMMENTS

_____

_____

@ SAFE HAVEN SOBRIETY

PERSONAL NOTES

PERSONAL

RELATIONS

SPIRITUAL

@ Safe Haven Sobriety

DAILY INVENTORY

Did I pray to know and follow God's will today?

What progress did I make?

What weaknesses do I need to surrender to God?

In what ways was I kind and loving?

Was I able to "let go and let God?"

Do I need to make amends to anyone?

Did faith or fear control my thoughts?

Am I taking care of myself physically, emotionally, and spiritually?

What am I grateful for today?

COMMENTS

@ Safe Haven Sobriety

PERSONAL NOTES

PERSONAL

RELATIONS

SPIRITUAL

@ SAFE HAVEN SOBRIETY

DAILY INVENTORY

Did I pray to know and follow God's will today?	

What progress did I make?	

What weaknesses do I need to surrender to God?	

In what ways was I kind and loving?	

Was I able to "let go and let God?"	

Do I need to make amends to anyone?	

Did faith or fear control my thoughts?	

Am I taking care of myself physically, emotionally, and spiritually?	

What am I grateful for today?	

COMMENTS

_____

_____

@ Safe Haven Sobriety

PERSONAL NOTES

PERSONAL

RELATIONS

SPIRITUAL

@ SAFE HAVEN SOBRIETY

DAILY INVENTORY

| Did I pray to know and follow God's will today? | |

| What progress did I make? | |

| What weaknesses do I need to surrender to God? | |

| In what ways was I kind and loving? | |

| Was I able to "let go and let God?" | |

| Do I need to make amends to anyone? | |

| Did faith or fear control my thoughts? | |

| Am I taking care of myself physically, emotionally, and spiritually? | |

| What am I grateful for today? | |

COMMENTS

@ Safe Haven Sobriety

PERSONAL NOTES

PERSONAL

RELATIONS

SPIRITUAL

@ SAFE HAVEN SOBRIETY

DAILY INVENTORY

Did I pray to know and follow God's will today?

What progress did I make?

What weaknesses do I need to surrender to God?

In what ways was I kind and loving?

Was I able to "let go and let God?"

Do I need to make amends to anyone?

Did faith or fear control my thoughts?

Am I taking care of myself physically, emotionally, and spiritually?

What am I grateful for today?

COMMENTS

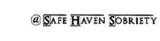

PERSONAL NOTES

PERSONAL

RELATIONS

SPIRITUAL

@ S̲AFE H̲AVEN S̲OBRIETY

DAILY INVENTORY

Did I pray to know and follow God's will today?

What progress did I make?

What weaknesses do I need to surrender to God?

In what ways was I kind and loving?

Was I able to "let go and let God?"

Do I need to make amends to anyone?

Did faith or fear control my thoughts?

Am I taking care of myself physically, emotionally, and spiritually?

What am I grateful for today?

COMMENTS

@ Safe Haven Sobriety

PERSONAL NOTES

PERSONAL

RELATIONS

SPIRITUAL

Manufactured by Amazon.ca
Bolton, ON